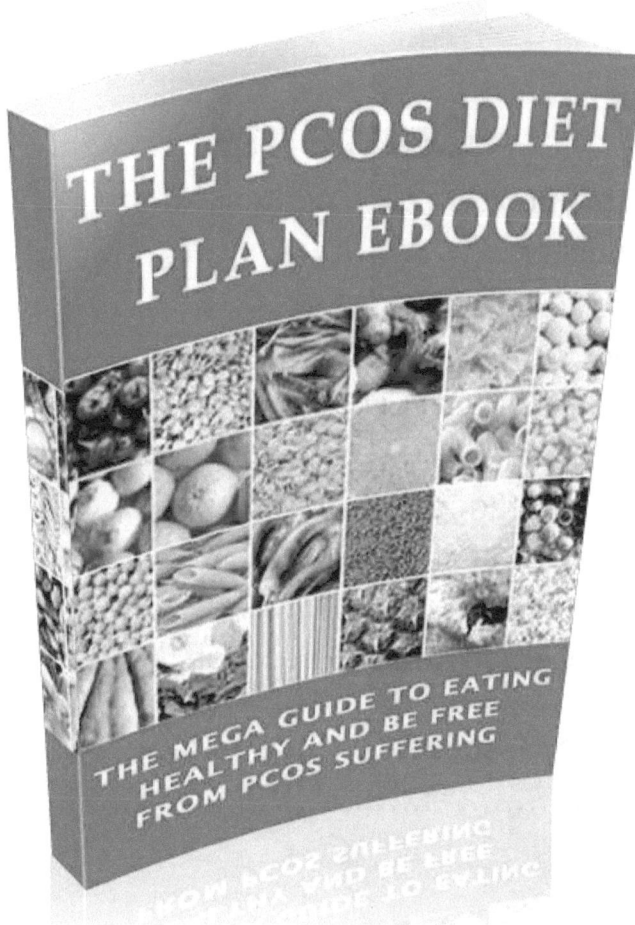

The PCOS Diet plan Ebook:
The Mega Guide to Eating Healthy
and be Free from PCOS Suffering

Contents

How to Use This Book

The PCOS Diet plan Ebook:The Mega Guide to Eating Healthy and be Free from PCOS Suffering; was written to assist PCOS patients who wish to manage their condition through proper diet and exercise. Polycystic ovarian syndrome is genetic in nature, and can be a chronic problem if left untreated.

This book is dedicated to all the brave women out there who wish to take back control of their bodies through intelligent planning and lifestyle modifications.

The book is divided into two distinct parts. Part 1: Introduction deals with the essential information regarding PCOS. If you wish to know more about this condition, I have prepared an informative overview in the section *Polycystic Ovarian Syndrome (PCOS).*

Information about the common symptoms of this disease can be found in *PCOS Symptoms.* For more information on what to expect when you visit your physician, read *Visiting a Doctor for the First Time.* If you are curious about the treatments available for PCOS, you can reference the section *General Treatment for PCOS.*

Part 2: The PCOS Diet deals with the complex and interrelated factors that come into play when designing a unique PCOS diet. For more information on the general principles of a sensible PCOS diet, read the section *General Principles of a PCOS Diet.* For advanced techniques on creating perfect meal plans, check out *Essential Strategies.* More advanced information can be found toward the end of the book.

Part 1: Introduction

My story begins on the year that I turned thirty-three. I had a great career in advertising, and I felt like I was on top of my game. I was earning well and, as a result, I partied and ate to my heart's desire.

Being single at that time, I didn't really care much about eating healthy, or even being healthy, for that matter. I just knew that I could do anything I wanted, anytime.

My feeling of superiority and immortality was brutally cut short when I began to experience strange symptoms. Hair began growing in places that shouldn't. I was fatigued most of the time, and I felt like my hormones were raging at all the wrong times of the month.

My monthly periods also became erratic and irregular. There were times when I menstruated only once every three months. As the symptoms persisted, I visited my doctor; after I described my symptoms, my doctor asked me to have a couple of tests performed.

It turned out that I had PCOS, or polycystic ovary syndrome. The name of the condition scared the living daylights out of me. I thought I was done for – until I noticed that my physician cracked a small smile when I began expressing my horror that I had PCOS.

My physician told me that, while PCOS may cause some severe problems if left untreated, a lot can be done to minimize its impact on my life.

That night I set out to find out as much as I could about my disease. What I learned about polycystic ovarian syndrome, or PCOS, really helped because I became familiar with what it was, and what it wasn't.

It has been many years since I began my journey towards becoming healthier. Within this period of challenges and, ultimately, personal healing, I married and had a wonderful daughter, Debra.

Like me, many PCOS patients dream of being able to battle the condition – and this book is all about winning in the battle against PCOS. I wrote this book with only one thing in mind: to help other PCOS patients who may not know where to start.

My other reason for writing this book was to carry out my advocacy of sensible and healthy eating. What you put into your body has a large impact on how it functions.

Eating is all about choices; no one is a victim, no one has been hoodwinked into eating something that they did not ultimately choose for themselves.

This is my lasting message to PCOS patients who feel that they have been somehow tricked into being unhealthy because they didn't know any better. Well, this is your ticket out of that trap. It's time to take back your life through strategic, healthy eating. Good luck!

Polycystic Ovarian Syndrome (PCOS)

Before you can properly wage war on PCOS and its symptoms, you have to first know what it is. The medical community believes that polycystic ovarian syndrome has a strong genetic component; this means that your risk of acquiring this condition is much higher if someone in your family has it.

Both males and females can carry the gene that triggers PCOS in women. So, this means that even if your mother doesn't have PCOS or the genes for it, you can still end up having PCOS if your father carries the gene. Your father will not exhibit any of the symptoms (for obvious reasons), but he can still pass it on to his female offspring.

PCOS is a very common health condition. Some diseases only have a one in a million chance of manifesting; PCOS has a one in fifteen in chance of occurring in women past the age of thirteen. That's right: once a girl reaches her teenage years, she already has a risk for developing PCOS.

When a woman has polycystic ovarian syndrome, her body has a tough time balancing her hormones. Hormones are chemical compounds in the human body that help regulate normal physiological processes.

Hormones affect the body at the cellular level, not just at the organ level. This is the main reason why hormonal problems tend to create a myriad of negative issues if they are left untreated.

Hormones have the ability to tell cells, tissues, and organs what to do, and how to behave. In short, hormones are power messenger agents that deliver specific messages, or orders, to parts of your body. When these messenger agents are firing off the wrong signals or commands, the body goes into disarray and imbalance.

Hormones are produced primarily by glands inside the body. The pituitary gland is one of the best examples of hormone-secreting tissues. Its sole job is to produce hormones that help regulate the normal growth and development of a person. If a person's pituitary gland is defective, a person may end up becoming too small or too tall (gigantism).

In the case of women who develop PCOS, the resulting hormonal imbalances brought about by this condition tend to trigger serious problems such as:

1. Difficulty in conceiving.

2. An increase in the total availability of the male sex hormone (also known as *androgen*).

3. The ovaries begin producing the male sex hormone as well as the female sex hormone (under normal, healthy circumstances the ovaries should never produce androgen at all).

4. Insulin resistance.

PCOS Symptoms

In order to differentiate PCOS from other types of conditions that produce hormonal imbalance, we must also be aware of the peculiar set of symptoms that are associated with this disease. Here is a breakdown of the common symptoms that arise when a woman develops polycystic ovarian syndrome:

1. Sudden eruption of *acne vulgaris*, or acne.

2. Inexplicable weight increase (not due to change in diet or exercise).

3. Inexplicable and sudden weight loss (again, not due to changes in your eating patterns or exercise regimen).

4. Male-pattern hair growth in the facial region, and in other parts of the body, such as the back and chest.

5. Inexplicable reduction of hair on the scalp (female balding).

6. Erratic menstrual pattern. A woman with PCOS may end up menstruating only once every two months or even less, depending on the severity of the hormonal imbalance and how her body is reacting to the disease.

7. Problems in getting pregnant (general fertility issues).

8. Some PCOS patients may also experience some degree of clinical depression as a result of having the symptoms, or because of the abnormal hormonal activity in the body.

Visiting a Doctor for the First Time

If you have any of the known symptoms of PCOS, the first step to the road to recovery is to visit your physician. Schedule an appointment as soon as possible, so your doctor can examine and confirm if your condition is indeed PCOS.

Remember: no amount of textual information can compare to the technical skill of a doctor. Do not try to self-diagnose if you have not been officially diagnosed as having PCOS. There are countless other health conditions out there that produce some, or almost all, of the symptoms of PCOS.

A definitive diagnosis is needed if you want to get the best treatment. If, in the end, you don't have PCOS, then at least you will have the benefit of knowing that your symptoms are being caused by some other condition, and you can begin planning your treatment options after getting your official diagnosis. Here are some things to expect when your doctor sees you for the first time:

1. He will be interested in your medical history, as well as your family's medical background. He will ask you if anyone in your immediate family has experienced the same symptoms.

   Note that even if you haven't the slightest clue if someone in your family has PCOS, your doctor will still be able to diagnose it with the help of medical tests.

2. One of the foundational procedures in ruling out other conditions is to perform a thorough physical examination.

   Your doctor will try to find out if you are developing abnormal hair growth patterns in places where you shouldn't have hair. Your body mass index (BMI), current weight, and your height will also be taken into consideration.

3. If you are underweight or overweight for your age and height that may be a key indicator that something might be wrong with your hormones. Another indicator that you may have PCOS is your blood pressure. Many PCOS patients have elevated blood pressure.

4. Checking your hormone levels is of utmost importance when diagnosing conditions such as PCOS; expect your doctor to request lab tests that will measure just how much estrogen and androgen you have in your body at the moment.

   Insulin resistance, blood glucose levels, etc., may also be measured, as PCOS has been known to trigger other metabolic conditions in the body.

General Treatment for PCOS

If you have already been diagnosed with polycystic ovarian syndrome, the parameters of your treatment will depend on how the syndrome is affecting your body and quality of life.

Your doctor will be your strongest ally when it comes to long-term management of this disease. Know that with the right treatment, your life will soon return to normal. A treatment plan for a PCOS patient will include one or all of the following elements:

1. PCOS diet and exercise routine that the patient can follow to improve her metabolism and quell any weight increases that may be slowly occurring due to hormonal imbalance.

2. Prescription medication to address the actual hormone imbalance in the body.

3. Additional medication for specific issues such as infertility.

Below are some important treatment guidelines that you should always remember if you want to get the upper hand in the battle against polycystic ovarian syndrome:

1. PCOS often gets worse if you don't care about what you eat, and how much physical activity you get in a day. Hormones influence the body's metabolism and hormonal imbalances (whether PCOS-related or not), often take place when your body is getting too many calories and is not burning off the right amount of energy every day.

I know that this might sound cliché, but I am going to repeat it anyway: start living a healthier life!

The basic information on how to achieve a healthier life is already public knowledge; unfortunately, many people still don't act upon this information (hence, the need for the multi-billion dollar fitness and health industry).

Don't worry: since you already have this book, you won't have to look anywhere else. We will be talking about diet and weight loss in detail later in the book.

2. Regular exercise is a top priority when you are trying to overcome PCOS. Exercise will help you achieve the following:

  a. Improved hormonal balance (this also applies to men who have health conditions that affect their hormone levels).

  b. Weight maintenance if your weight is still in the normal range.

  c. Weight loss if your weight has increased significantly because of PCOS.

  d. Natural detoxification of the body.

  e. Reduction of water retention due to a sedentary lifestyle and, in some cases, too much sodium in one's diet.

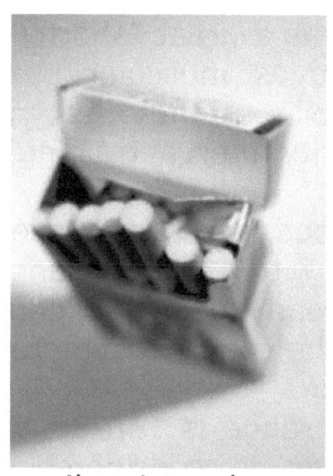

Smoking can cause spikes in androgen levels in the body, leading to further hormone imbalance. Additionally, there is a strong link between regular tobacco use and various cancers and heart diseases.

There are two types of exercise that you should integrate into your own fitness regimen. The first category is *steady-state physical activity.*

This includes walking, jogging, using the Stair Master, running, cycling, indoor biking, etc. These exercises improve blood circulation and overall oxygen availability in the tissues, so the more you do them, the more efficient you become in exercising.

The muscular fatigue and exhaustion that is common when a person exercises for the first time will gradually dissipate as you continue to exercise regularly.

The second category of exercise is *high intensity interval training.* The principles of HIIT can be applied to different forms of exercise. HIIT should be employed to improve your body's endurance and metabolism.

It is also viewed as a great "shortcut" to better health, because it improves muscular strength, speed, and muscular adaptability greatly. Ask your physical trainer about high intensity interval training!

3. Monitor your blood pressure closely after you have been diagnosed with PCOS. Chances are your blood pressure had already been "spiking" even before you started noticing the common symptoms of PCOS.

   The high-normal range is 130/80. Anything above the high-normal range is considered hypertension. The great thing about this situation is that there are so many prescription medications available in the market that deal with your type of condition.

   If one prescription drug doesn't work well with your body's chemistry, you can always ask your doctor for an alternative prescription.

4. If your weight has been increasing steadily these past few months, it is definitely time to start shedding those excess pounds.

   According to medical literature, shedding between 10-15 pounds of excess body weight can help reverse the symptoms of PCOS. Additionally, other bodily maladies related to being overweight will also be addressed when you shed weight.

5. Tobacco use exacerbates PCOS. Scientific research shows that women who regularly smoke tend to have much higher male hormone levels than women who don't use tobacco. Androgen is the male sex hormone that causes hirsutism (male-pattern hair growth on the body and face) and other PCOS-related symptoms.

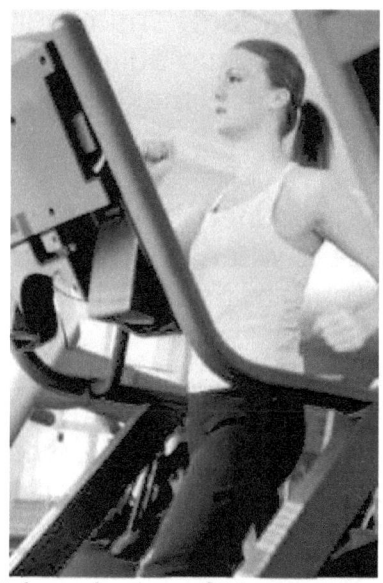

Exercise is considered one of the most effective ways to rebalance the body's hormone levels. Try it today!

Part 2: The PCOS Diet

Healthy Eating Defined

A PCOS diet, unlike other fad diets out there, does not require special shakes, powders, and other strange additions to one's diet. There is no magic bullet involved and, for the most part, you will be the one making all the magic in your daily diet.

Since there is no magic bullet or wonder cure, the placebo effect is definitely absent when you start on a diet that aims to alleviate the symptoms of polycystic ovarian syndrome.

This part of the book deals with the many guidelines that will help you create your very own PCOS diet. That's right – I'm not going to give you a strict meal plan. I believe that in order for a diet to become permanent and effective, it must be planned and modified by the person using it.

Strict diets may work for a short period of time, but looking at the current "rebound" statistics (or people who gain weight again after trying a diet for a few months), it's safe to say that modifying a diet according to your evolving needs is a much better option.

So again, I'm not going to say things like "you can only eat a cup of peas and some cheese at lunch". I want you to create your own PCOS diet based on sound principles and factual information we have right now about the disease.

This way, you will become much more adept with what you eat. In the end, your expertise with the PCOS diet will help you achieve weight loss and fitness goals, too.

General Principles of a PCOS Diet

A PCOS diet does not have a strict form; anyone can create a good PCOS diet based on sound, scientific principles. Here are the essential principles of an effective PCOS diet that you should always keep in mind:

I. Portion Control

A portion is defined as a specific serving size of any kind of food or beverage. It is a measure of how much food you are eating at any one time.

A serving size can be defined in two ways. It can be the amount of food that can be used to understand the caloric content and nutritional value of a specific food item, and it can also refer to the recommended quantity of food every time you eat.

For example, the recommended serving size for bread is 1 to 2 slices per meal only. A single serving, or 1 slice of white, sliced bread contains about 85 kcal of energy.

Each kind of food has a definite serving size. The serving sizes of foods and beverages are often set forth by the United States Department of Agriculture (USDA).

A serving size can also be set forth by food manufacturers. Both standards can be used to understand the caloric and nutritional content of the food or beverage that you wish to examine.

PCOS patients should be aware of what "1 serving" actually means when they eat different kinds of food. For example, if you reach for a bag of chocolate chip cookies, do you know what "1 serving" really means?

Check the back of the package (the nutritional label), and you will see: one serving does *not* mean the whole bag or how much you can eat in one sitting!

To illustrate just how easily people can get confused about serving sizes, let me tell you a story about a good friend of mine who wanted to lose weight.

She was overweight most of her life and by the time she hit her thirties she had developed high blood pressure and was already showing signs of pre-diabetes.

In short, she had to do something about her eating if she wanted to quell the health problems that she had. The first thing that she did was to look for healthy snacks to replace the myriad of chocolate bars and candies she regularly stocked at home. She succeeded in finding stuff made from oatmeal and wholegrain. Many of the things that she did find *were* healthy... if they were eaten in moderation.

When I visited my friend a few weeks after she started her new crusade to become healthier, I found her munching on a large bag of what appeared to be butter-flavored oatmeal cookies.

I asked her immediately "how much of that stuff have you been eating?" She replied proudly "I've been eating one serving every day." I was confused for a few seconds until it hit me: she thought that 1 serving was one whole bag of cookies!

She showed me the nutritional label at the back of the cookie package. The nutritional label read "1 serving = 104 calories." What she failed to see was the line of text underneath: *total servings – 25.*

When I explained to her what a serving really meant, the color drained from her face. Because she didn't know any better, she had ended up consuming an additional 2,600 calories every day since she started. Since then, my friend had become more aware of serving sizes. She never wanted to repeat the same dire mistake twice!

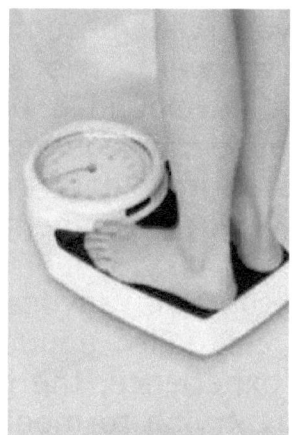

Sensible weight loss can help reduce the symptoms of PCOS in the <u>long-term.</u>

II.   Counting Calories Matter

I am aware that there is a vocal crusade against counting calories in the weight loss market. But, the truth of the matter is that if you do not know how to count calories *at all*, there is no way for you to know how many calories you are consuming at any one time.

Counting calories is more than just a mechanical process of limiting yourself whenever you eat. Nowadays, caloric information about any kind of food often comes with a breakdown of its nutrients.

When you exert a lot of effort in discovering how many calories there are in the foods that you commonly eat, you also gain knowledge about the components of the food, such as how much it contains of protein, carbohydrates, sugars, etc.

In short, you will become an expert in food composition as well. It is unfortunate that calorie counting has developed a bad reputation over the decades because of misguided "diet experts" who are more interested in selling "quick fixes" than helping people lose weight permanently.

Many diet programs advocate calorie counting so people will feel guilty about eating certain things. Well, in my experience, the guilt doesn't help at all. When you are trying to modify your eating patterns the last thing you need is guilt over the foods that you want to eat.

What I want you to develop is a special diet IQ that will help you decide which foods are best for you, *based on your needs and current diet parameters.*

For example, let us say that you were eating 2,800 calories before, and you want to lose 10 pounds of extra body weight.

You can do this easily by cutting 500 to 800 calories off your daily intake. You will then be left with 2,000 calories (give or take a few hundred).

How will you be "spending" those calories? Without knowledge of the actual number of calories in food, it would be impossible to hit your target.

For example, did you know that a single serving of a chocolate bar can contain as many as 250 calories? And that a regular cheese burger from McDonalds contains roughly 500 calories from sugar and fat?

Intelligent calorie counting is a necessity in today's world, because food and beverage manufacturers are finding increasingly creative ways to make their products less healthy and more calorie-laden than before.

III. Stick to the Basics of a Heart-Healthy Diet

One of the direst consequences of having PCOS is an increased risk of developing high blood pressure, and other heart conditions.

In our day and age, where processed foods and fast food junk are the kings and queens of homes, schools, and offices, it is *hard* to avoid food items that can cause your blood pressure to shoot up.

The only solution to this problem is to become even more mindful of what you actually eat. The medical community agrees that, in order to cut down your total risk for blocked arteries, you need to reduce the amount of fat you are consuming.

This information has been around since the seventies. However, new information suggests that it's not really fat, per se, that is to blame, but the kind of fat you are consuming.

Additionally, it has been discovered that too many simple carbohydrates in a person's diet can be equally lethal in terms of triggering high blood pressure and metabolic issues, like diabetes.

With all this confusing information, where should a PCOS patient do? Should she eat more fat? Less fat? In my own studies of weight loss and healthy eating, I have found the following guidelines extremely helpful in maintaining my own weight, and cutting down my risk for diabetes and heart problems:

➢ Animal fat is definitely out of the question. Animal fat contains too many calories and is high in LDL or low-density lipoproteins. LDL blocks arteries and also increases inflammation in the body.

Definitely not good for someone who is at risk for high blood pressure! So, when you are eating pork or beef, be sure to eat only lean cuts of meat, and please remove all the visible fat.

You will still be consuming some fat, but most of the fat in the serving of meat will be physically removed. If you see fat, just slice it off and throw it away.

The flavor of the meat is in the muscle tissue, not in the fat. Another reason why you should avoid eating animal fat is the fact that animals (like humans) store a significant amount of toxins (including heavy metals) in fat.

It's a way for their bodies to limit the impact of these toxins on the overall physiology of the animal. The toxins stay in the fat tissues indefinitely.

When an animal is slaughtered for meat, the toxins are not drained away just because the animal is dead. The toxins remain in the fat tissue, and they aren't removed by cooking, either. These toxins are not detectable by sight, smell, or taste, which makes them even more insidious to one's health.

➢ Not all fat is evil. In fact, if you stick to healthy oils, like olive oil and fish oil, you are actually doing your heart a world of good.

Natural fat from fish contains omega 3 fatty acids. Omega 3 fatty acids help reduce inflammation in the body, and have been proven to be protective of the heart and blood vessels.

Olive oil and other natural vegetable oils also have heart-healthy benefits. There is a caveat though – anything in excess is still bad for the body.

Drizzling a bit of olive oil over a large quantity of salad that is low in salt is perfectly fine. Deep-frying large quantities of chicken in olive oil does *not* reduce calories, or their inherent negative impact on the body.

Additionally, using too much oil (of any kind) can increase your body weight because of the extra calories. A single tablespoon of oil can pack as much as 100 kcal. That's how energy-dense oil is (ever wondered why used cooking oil can be used in diesel engines?).

➢ Watch your carbohydrates, as too many carbs in your diet can also cause metabolic problems. We will be talking about this in detail later on.

IV. Keep Alcohol at Bay

It's no secret that alcohol still has a powerful grip on both men and women, especially when it comes to social gatherings.

Unfortunately, some people develop a chemical dependence on alcohol, making it nearly impossible for them to lay off the beer or hard drinks for long periods of time.

If you drink regularly, it's time to reduce your consumption to just one serving *per day*. That's one bottle for beer, a small glass of wine and, if you really have to, a small shot glass of hard liquor. There are so many reasons why alcohol is bad for a person with polycystic ovarian syndrome:

> ➢ Alcoholic beverages contain lots of calories. A single bottle of beer contains about 150 calories of carbohydrates (sugars), and not much else.

> Though some people are championing wine and beer as potential heart savers, it still remains a fact that only a miniscule percentage of the population drinks beer or any kind of alcoholic beverage for their therapeutic effects.

> Most folks just drink to get smashed and happily drunk. See the problem here? It is very easy to abuse alcohol, because almost anyone can buy them from any corner store in any town or city.

> When alcohol enters a person's body, it produces two very distinct effects: elevated blood pressure, and constricted blood vessels.

As you may already know, elevated blood pressure can cause stroke or heart attacks. Constricted blood vessels, on the other hand, increase a person's risk for cardiovascular anomalies.

So, if you think about it really hard, the risks associated with drinking too much are really not worth it because, in the end, it will be your body that would be taking 100% of the chemical impact of the beverage.

> Too much alcohol increases the deposition of fat in the belly region. A large belly almost always means that you have more visceral fat clinging close to your organs.

Visceral fat isn't *just* body fat. Studies have shown that too much visceral fat can be damaging to one's health.

It appears that visceral fat produces chemical byproducts that promote inflammation. Having a higher percentage of visceral fat can also increase your risk for diabetes and heart disease.

➢ Current research shows that alcohol has a detrimental impact on the natural hormonal balance of the body. If you have already been diagnosed with PCOS, drinking too much alcohol might be pounding new nails into your coffin.

Stopping alcohol, on the other hand, will definitely help restore your hormone levels to normal. Stopping a persistent alcohol habit may not be the known cure for PCOS, but at the very least you will have the advantage of *not* contributing to your existing hormonal issues.

Essential Strategies

Earlier in this part of the book, I mentioned that I was not interested in laying down any dogmatic parameters for your own PCOS diet. I want *you* to determine the course of your diet modification, based on sound principles.

This way, you can go about the change in your diet (and lifestyle) at a pace that is comfortable for you. Your comfort and happiness level during the transition period is of utmost importance.

Normally, people go about it backwards: they start with a very strict plan, and they adjust their routines and emotions around this plan. More often than not, this approach produces ruthless backlashes and diet rebounds that don't help at all.

To avoid the common trap of being forced into a strict mold within a short period of time, we are going to do it differently. Instead of asking you to follow very precise steps, I am going to describe to you what an effective PCOS diet is.

You are free to do your own research, and to create your own meal plans, based on your available time and resources. You will have the freedom of taking as little or as much as you want from the book.

As long as you do not do something that is obviously against established principles (e.g. drinking too much alcohol, even if you know that can be detrimental to your condition), every bit of effort that you exert in creating and implementing a new PCOS diet is considered legitimate. Sound good? Let us begin!

I. Watch What You Drink

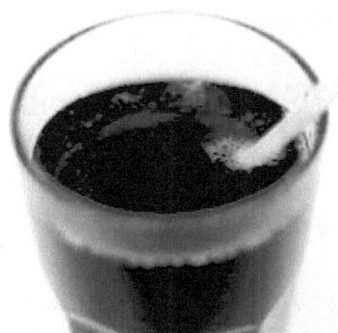

Diet softdrinks often contain caffeine and artificial sweeteners that are equally harmful to the body's natural chemistry.

One of the biggest mistakes that people make when they are trying to eat healthier is to begin consuming beverages like diet softdrinks and energy drinks on a regular basis.

While it is true that these beverages do not add a heap of calories to your diet, we should all remember that they are not health drinks, and they are not even organic.

Energy drinks might taste good, and many of them actually have fewer than 100 calories per serving. However, energy drinks provide that "buzz" to its drinkers because of caffeine.

Caffeine is not recommended for PCOS sufferers, because it directly affects a person's blood pressure. And, as you may already know, PCOS patients have a higher risk for developing high blood pressure than folks who do not have PCOS and other similar hormonal problems.

Additionally, energy drinks and low calorie drinks have high levels of artificial sweeteners, like aspartame and sodium. Sodium is another common culprit when it comes to elevated blood pressure.

Some people with hypertension develop a severe sensitivity to sodium. This means they really have to cut down on their sodium intake if they want to regulate their blood pressure levels.

Otherwise, they will be faced with sudden spikes of high blood pressure that will put them in the direct path of stroke, heart attack, and even deep vein thrombosis (vascular blockages).

Now, some of you might be wondering: if diet sodas and energy drinks are out of the question, what about sports drinks, like Gatorade? Can you drink Gatorade with impunity, since is is recommended for athletes and fitness buffs? Not necessarily.

A regular bottle of orange-flavored Gatorade contains about 130 calories from added sugar. So, from the caloric content alone, it is not really a good choice for PCOS patients. You can get the equivalent amount of energy from something more nutritious, like salad with light dressing, or even a piece of fruit.

This point really characterizes what we are trying to do when we are designing a PCOS diet. We want the body to receive not only an adequate amount of calories for daily work, but also a significant amount of vitamins, minerals, carbohydrates, proteins, and good fats, so that it will continue functioning normally.

And here's the thing: beverages with artificial sweeteners, such as aspartame, may seem harmless but in reality, these beverages are actually messing with your internal hormonal balance as well.

Recent studies show that even if aspartame is *not* a form of carbohydrate, it can still affect your metabolism in general. So, what can you drink in place of all these artificially sweetened, calorie-laden beverages?

I have just one word for you: *water.* Start with the simplest and *best* form of hydration for the body: pure water.

Drink it warm or cold, it doesn't matter; just make sure that it's water. I am not advocating fancy filtering systems, nor am I telling people to buy water systems that adjust the acidity of water.

I am just telling fellow PCOS patients to go back to the basics, and start drinking more water. Common knowledge states that we need to drink about eight glasses of water every day. There is nothing wrong with this adage.

If it seems too much, then chances are you probably don't drink that much water throughout the day. Start drinking more water, and you will see a big difference in how you feel. Of course, if your doctor tells you to limit your fluids because of severe high blood pressure, then heed his warning.

But if are allowed to drink as much as you want, then drink your fill of water. Of course, only the brave few will be able to stick to pure water every day.

I'm sure many of you will be thinking of a soda pretty soon... And I'm not judging you for that either. What I do suggest is to reduce the quantity of artificially flavored beverages you are consuming on a daily basis, in favor of pure water.

This is where true change starts. There is no need to shock your system by eliminating all of a sudden the beverages that you have been drinking for many years. However, bear in mind that if change doesn't start now, it is unlikely that it will ever begin. So start small, but initiate the change *now.*

II. Consider Carbohydrate Reduction

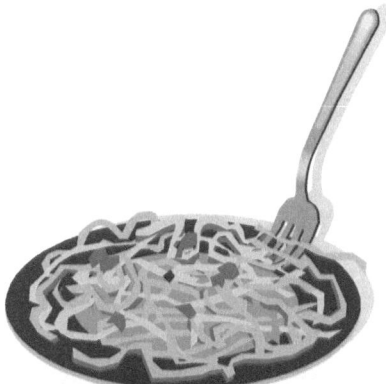

Many people consume hundreds of grams of carbohydrates without noticing it... Changing this picture may spell the difference between aggravating PCOS and relief from its most severe symptoms.

Under normal circumstances, a person will function fairly well with a diet that is 50% carbohydrates (the remaining 50% would be comprised of fat, protein, fiber, etc.).

However, in the case of women who have PCOS, the opposite might be true: a reduction in carbohydrate intake just might make a PCOS patient's life that much better.

Before we delve into the technical details of why carbohydrate reduction just might help you live a fuller and less problematic life with PCOS, let us review what carbohydrates are in the first place.

Carbohydrates are micronutrients used by the body primarily for fuel. They are an organic compound and, when they enter the body through a meal, carbohydrates are broken down by the body into a form that is immediately usable: glucose.

Glucose is used by the muscles for energy, and is also used to normalize countless physiological processes. Carbohydrates are the primary fuel that drives the human body.

In fact, the human brain requires glucose in order to function normally. This is probably one of the biggest reasons why people have a tough time kick-starting their work in the office if they haven't eaten anything in the morning.

The brain is literally starving for some glucose. And since lunchtime is still some hours away, the fatigued, sleepy feeling will remain unless the person eats something to fuel his lethargic brain.

Now, there are two general categories of carbohydrates in the human diet. The first one is called *simple carbohydrates.* Simple carbohydrates are represented by stuff like refined sugar, fruit sugars, etc.

Simple carbohydrates are easily digested and absorbed by the human body, and they have a tendency to rapidly increase blood glucose levels.

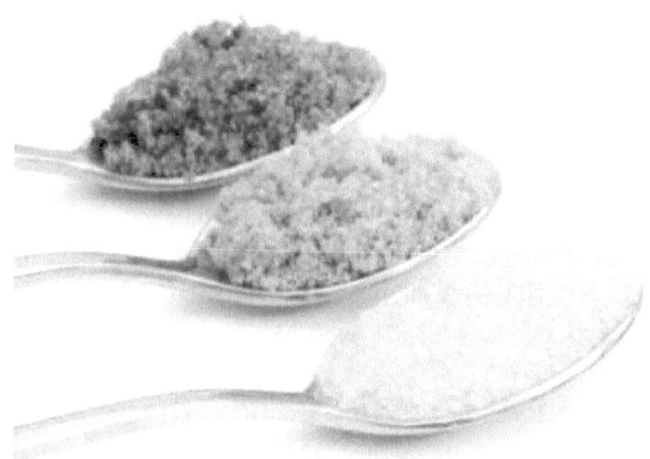

Refined sugars should be limited in a PCOS diet, because they provide very little nutritive value and far too many calories in every serving.

Nowadays, food manufacturers use simple carbohydrate sources like HFCS (high fructose corn syrup). These sweeteners are cheap to produce and are packed with more sugar calories than you can imagine.

On the other side of the ring are complex carbohydrates, like rolled oatmeal. Complex carbohydrates are not easily broken down by the body.

So, when you eat food that is rich in complex carbohydrates, you feel fuller for a longer period of time, and your blood glucose level remains stable, for the most part. Some of you might be thinking: only old and frail people need complex carbohydrates!

Well, think again: the best bodybuilders and athletes in the world *prefer* complex carbohydrates, because they release energy in a staggered manner.

People with high-energy requirements tend to consume higher quantities of complex carbohydrates, so they will have more energy all day long. No fitness buff worth his title would say that he would prefer a Snickers bar to complex carbs.

That's because candies and other junk foods filled with sugars (a type of simple carb) don't provide sufficient energy over longer periods of time.

Think of carbohydrates as fuel for a fire. When you consume simple carbs, you throw most of your wood chips into the fire to create a massive blaze (this is the spike in your blood sugar level).

After a few minutes, the blaze dissipates and, eventually, you have a tiny fire in front of you (or the first is extinguished altogether). The story is different with complex carbohydrates.

With complex carbohydrates, you won't be throwing all your fuel into the fire. Instead, you will only be using a small quantity of fuel to throw into the fire to keep it going.

The fire will not transform into a massive blaze, but it will keep burning, and the size of the fire will be consistent. The process itself is repeated until the fuel is completely exhausted. Do you see the difference now?

With complex carbohydrates, your body will receive a much more consistent amount of energy for its daily needs. This is the main reason why doctors and nutritionists advocate whole grains: because these are the most readily available sources of complex carbohydrates.

Now that you are familiar with what carbohydrates are and what they do in the body, let us go back to the main issue at hand: carbohydrate reduction. If carbohydrates are so important to the body, then why must we reduce our intake of carbohydrates?

The answer to this question is actually quite complex and admittedly, needs to be considered on a case-to-case basis.

Carbohydrate reduction, *in general*, will be able to help a person regulate his hormones because, this way, insulin resistance will be reduced and blood glucose levels will also be restored (if the patient is medicating for such a condition as well).

Current medical studies that center on the effects of a carbohydrate-reduced diet indicate that people who cut their carbohydrate intake to just 20 grams per day lost an average of twelve pounds of total body weight in just half a year.

There are other factors that come into play, but one thing is for sure: the weight loss for the respondents occurred when they agreed to take on the challenge of consuming only 20 grams of carbohydrates a day.

After half a year of religiously maintaining a low-carb diet, the respondents (who were all women) were examined using standard medical tests.

The results were promising: 100% respondents lost no less than twelve pounds of body weight. Additionally, the insulin resistance, that was present in all of the respondents, was reduced greatly.

Here's another bit of good news for PCOS patients who are already suffering from fertility problems: in the same study, a handful of women also became pregnant as they were cutting down their carbohydrate intake.

I know for a fact that the emotional toll of PCOS increases greatly when a woman is unable to conceive, because she has hormonal imbalances. Reducing your carbohydrate intake just might solve one of PCOS's worst effects: infertility, or the inability to conceive.

III. Balance the Equation with Protein

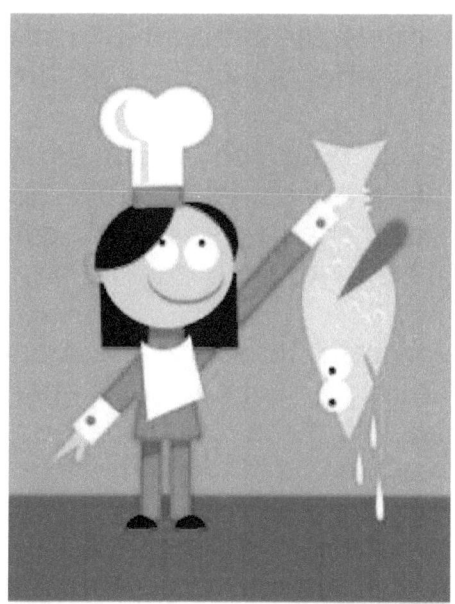

Fish is one of the leanest and most nutritious sources of dietary protein, which is pre-requisite if you want to build lean muscle mass for increased metabolism.

In the previous discussion, we explored in depth what could potentially happen to *you* if you drastically reduced your carbohydrate intake every day.

Note that you must consult with your doctor prior to implementing this massive change in your diet, because if you already have metabolic issues, you may not be able to tide over the rough transition period that follows the reduction.

An average adult consumes more than 100 grams of carbohydrates per day. 20 grams of carbohydrates is really a miniscule amount of carbs, and may cause severe side effects like nausea, dizziness, etc.

As always, your physician is your number one partner when it comes to your health. *Do not* make any drastic changes without consulting with your doctor! This is for your safety, primarily.

That being said, let's talk about another diet strategy that just might help you permanently quell issues that arise from having too much glucose in your bloodstream.

We all know that PCOS can aggravate diabetes, and pre-diabetics should be prepared for any sudden changes in their body's chemistry.

If you are pre-diabetic/diabetic and you have also been diagnosed with PCOS, it is essential that you attain normal fasting blood sugar levels *and* a fitter body. By *fit,* I really mean you should keep your weight within normal range through sensible eating and regular exercise.

And this is my cue to introduce to you the value of protein, when you are already implementing a carbohydrate-reduced diet.

Protein is the building block of muscle tissue, and is also used by the body for many chemical processes. Without sufficient protein, you won't be able to build lean muscle mass, and this can really hamper your body's natural ability to raise its basal metabolic rate. More muscle mass means more fire (figuratively) to burn extra calories.

When your basal metabolic rate increases, your body literally becomes a fat-burning machine. But, in order for your body to become truly conditioned to become a fat burning machine, you need to give it enough protein.

Advanced studies in sports fitness indicate that, if a person's diet is about 30% protein, body fat would progressively drop as the person's lean muscle mass increases.

This astounding transformation will only be possible *if* you are also able to regulate your carbohydrate intake. I cannot emphasize this enough: if you are working out all day, but you are unable to cut your carbohydrate intake, the weight loss and the lean muscle mass that you want will be slow in coming.

Excess carbohydrates in the body are transformed into fat, which explains why carbohydrate lovers often pack more pounds in a shorter period of time than folks who eat low or moderate amounts of carbohydrates on a daily basis.

Carbohydrates, like fat, are a concentrated form of energy, so it is best to consume them in moderation, regardless of your current health condition.

At this point in time, you may already be thinking of modifying your diet to introduce more protein and fewer sources of simple carbohydrates, and you may also be thinking of what particular sources of protein are best for weight maintenance or weight loss.

Of course, you will have a tougher time looking for healthy choices when you eat out, so I would suggest that you cook most of your meals at home. It takes more time and effort but, in the end, you will be glad that you opted for home-cooked meals.

Home-cooked meals provide absolute control in terms of what actually goes into your body during breakfast, lunch, snack time, and dinner.

Two protein sources stand out in terms of practicality and nutritive value: lean beef and lean cuts of chicken. Your cooking methods also matter.

Roasted and stewed dishes are best for weight loss. Avoid frying meat, as this greatly increases the fat content of the meat.

Roasting helps drain fat, naturally; stewing, on the other hand, can help give you that feeling of fullness without necessarily adding to the total target calories. Stewing is also great if you are hesitant about eating vegetables.

When vegetables are stewed in a tasty sauce, they taste just like the meat, and you will probably chow down on the veggies with little anxiety or hesitation.

A Primer on Carbohydrate Reduction & Other PCOS Diet Parameters

As you may have already noticed, one of the foundations of an effective PCOS diet is carbohydrate reduction. It's not for everyone, but for the purpose of lessening the impact of PCOS, it is generally recommended that PCOS patients reduce their carbohydrate intake at least a little, to see results quickly.

Carbohydrates can increase a person's weight in a matter of months, if things get out of hand, and the resulting fat deposition (especially in the belly area) can make hormone balance restoration much more difficult.

Reducing your overall carbohydrate intake can be tough, so I have taken the liberty of devoting a specific section to this crucial step.

Note that this section also covers other interrelated topics as well, so if things get a little confusing at times, just take notes and combine the ideas later on.

1. Insulin resistance is probably the number one concern of physicians who have been tasked with managing the health of a PCOS patient. The human body is dependent on normal hormonal balance when it comes to breaking down glucose and maintaining normal glucose levels.

When hormonal balance goes haywire, insulin resistance can develop. Over a long stretch, insulin resistance can mean type 2 diabetes, which can bring a whole new set of problems. If you want to avoid this scenario completely, you have to plan your new diet as soon as possible.

In my years of research, one of the most effective formulas I have seen is the high fiber plus low carbohydrate diet. Again, I am not stating this as a dogma, but rather as a guiding principle only.

Some people are not allowed to consume large quantities of dietary fiber because of chronic flatulence and other related health conditions.

The same applies to low glycemic or low carbohydrate diets: they shouldn't be taken lightly, and any changes to a person's diet should always be monitored by a certified health professional.

2. Our natural hormone levels can be affected by chemicals and preservatives in the food and beverages that we consume. To lessen the impact of these chemicals on your own health, it is best to stick to organic food products and beverages.

Yes, organic is often more expensive and is harder to find, *but* it is your body that we are talking about here. The extra bucks that you pay for organic food will be translated to better health in the future.

Think of it as just paying for a healthier body. If people can pay $300 or more for a new used car, shouldn't people be willing to spend even more for their own bodies?

3. If you have been dependent on processed food items and fast food for many decades, it might be a good idea to engage in a raw food cleanse.

   Raw food cleanses have been around for years and, while it isn't exactly rocket science, an organic cleanse just might be what the doctor ordered. Ask your doctor first if a raw food cleanse is a good idea, before engaging in one.

   If you get a green light from your doctor, stick to fresh fruits and vegetables *only* for at least seven days. As for beverages, do not allow yourself to drink anything else but pure, clean water.

   The benefits of a raw food cleanse are myriad, but what I want you to really achieve is freedom (if only partially) from processed foods and too many carbohydrates in your diet.

   By engaging in an organic cleanse like the raw food cleanse, you will be giving your body a chance to rest and recuperate. During this time your kidneys and liver will also be getting some much needed rest.

   After seven days, I recommend gently easing out of the cleanse by eating small quantities of regular food. This transition period can take up to three days, depending on how long you chose to cleanse yourself internally.

Do not chow down on French fries and hamburgers after the seventh day! Eating large quantities of regular food immediately after a cleanse can cause digestive problems and, trust me, you will not like what may follow if you force your body to start processing regular food again in a very abrupt manner.

After cleansing your system for seven days, you will notice a big change in how you feel, and you will probably have no trouble at all easing into another diet modification plan (e.g. carbohydrate restriction during mealtimes).

4. Controlling your weight doesn't mean you have to skip meals. On the contrary, you have to start eating *more* if you want to take control of your body. In the world of PCOS management and weight loss, *frequency* is the genie in the lamp.

   You need to eat more often than usual to really fire up the metabolism engine. Some people eat only twice a day (big lunch and big supper), and while these people might say that they are fine not eating breakfast, they are actually harming their bodies severely.

   Breakfast is indeed the most important meal of the day, because what you eat for breakfast actually sets the tune of your whole day. If you give your body lots of empty calories during breakfast, your body will crave empty calories until dinnertime.

If you don't eat breakfast at all, your body will send confusing signals to your brain during lunch and dinner. You will end up eating more than what is sensible for your age and height, because your body's internal hunger/satiation meter is not functioning properly.

How many times should a PCOS patient eat in a day? According to experienced dietitians, the best formula would be three square meals a day *and* three small snacks.

Portion control should be implemented every step of the way. You must not fall into the trap of noshing on unhealthy things during snack time, or during dinner time.

Some people find it difficult not to overeat at night because they have felt deprived the whole day. I ask you to practice utmost self-control, especially at dinnertime, because it is very easy to overeat.

An extra plate of pasta or meatballs can make a person's caloric intake jump from 2,000 calories to 2,500 calories easily.

5. One of the easiest ways to implement a low carbohydrate diet is by reading and remembering the basic GI (glycemic index) values of common food items.

The glycemic index is a measure of how quickly a serving of food (or beverage) can increase a blood glucose level of a person. Below are some examples of low glycemic index food items and their GI values *per serving*:

Low GI foods:

➢ *Banana bread*

➢ *Banana cake*

➢ *Regular apples*

➢ *Oranges*

➢ *Barley bread*

➢ *Whole grain white bread*

➢ *Tortillas (made from corn)*

➢ *Tortillas (made from wheat)*

➢ *Fresh tomato juice*

➢ *Freshly squeezed orange juice*

➢ *Bran products*

- Rolled oatmeal (instant or quick-cook)

- Barley

- Quinoa grain

- Brown rice

- Bulgur

- Sugar-reduced ice cream

- Dates

- Grapefruit

- Fresh pears

- Peanuts

- Blackeyed peas

- Kidney beans

- Red beans

- Yellow beans

- White beans

- Tofu

- Soy based products (with the exception of flavored soy milk with added refined sugar)

➢ Macaroni (manufactured from wheat)

➢ Parsnips

➢ Protein shakes

➢ Yogurt

➢ Fruit yogurt

➢ Greek yogurt

➢ Fruit smoothies made from soy

➢ Prunes

➢ Raisins

➢ Butter bean

➢ Lentils

➢ Mung beans

➢ Cashew nuts

➢ Vermicelli

➢ M&M chocolate candy with peanuts

➢ Low fat milk

➢ Organic yams

➢ Taro root

The foods that I have just listed down have a glycemic index of 55 or less. These food items are considered the best options when you are looking for food that won't strain your body's ability to break down carbohydrates and control blood sugar levels.

By just going through the list you will begin to see patterns in the GI values. For example, did you notice that most beans have a low GI rating? That means you can eat more beans without worrying about the random blood sugar spikes, because they are low GI food items.

6. A truly effective PCOS diet will not leave you feeling starved and hungry for junk food. Sure, there might be some resistance on your part when you are just starting out with this type of diet.

Most of the resistance that you will be experiencing will be stemming from your own mind because, admittedly, it is hard to change one's long standing eating patterns.

To facilitate your shift from your usual diet to your new PCOS diet, it is absolutely essential that you strike a balance between the three major macronutrients. You need fat, protein, *and* a small amount of carbohydrates in order to keep your body satisfied with your new meals.

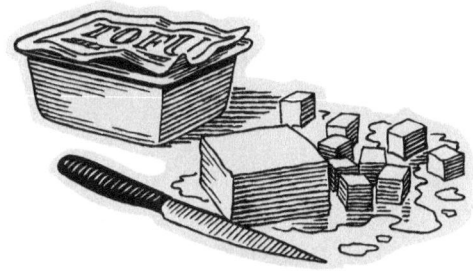

*Soy products such as tofu are excellent sources of protein –
they can be your "go to" when you are looking for satisfying
low glycemic index food items.*

7. If you are tired of eating beef and chicken, then it
   might be a great time to start exploring the undersea
   world for more delectable protein sources.

   Most wild-caught fish such as salmon is wonderful for
   PCOS patients because of the high protein and high fat
   content of the fish. Don't get me wrong: the fat in fish
   is very different from fat found in pork, beef, and
   chicken.

   As I have mentioned before, the oil found in fish is
   actually good for your heart, and will *not* exacerbate
   the symptoms of PCOS. Fish oil is a top-notch option if
   you want to introduce more omega 3 fatty acids into
   your diet.

If you are having a tough time taking omega 3 supplements, opt for a more natural route: eat more fish! Three to four servings of fish a week can help reduce your BMI, and may also help keep your heart healthier.

We place special emphasis on your cardiovascular system because patients with PCOS have a much higher risk for heart problems than women who do not have PCOS.

It is very important that you take good care of your heart, because it will take a beating if you don't pay attention to the basic of cardiovascular health.

8. I know that cutting one's carbohydrate intake to just twenty grams per day can be impossible for many women. I also know that, for the most part, you will be negotiating the fine line between maintaining a normal life and managing your condition.

You don't need additional stress just because you want to take control of PCOS through your diet. If you want to reduce your carbohydrate intake, it is best to aim for an attainable median line.

So, if you want an ideal target that won't make your head ache, try gunning for 120 grams of total carbohydrates per day.

To give you an idea as to how many carbohydrates you can have before you reach 120 grams, let us assume that you will only be eating white bread for the whole day.

One slice of wheat bread contains 23 grams of carbohydrates. If you are limited to wheat bread the whole day, you can eat 5.2 slices of bread before reaching the 120-gram limit.

If we change the scenario a bit and substitute macaroni (43 grams of carbs/serving), you can eat up to 2.7 servings of macaroni easily before going over the 120-gram limitation.

9. Having a great breakfast is pre-requisite to having a good metabolism throughout the day. Unfortunately, many people get stuck when it comes to deciding what they should eat in the morning.

If we were to circle back just a bit, you will remember that it is important to strike a balance between the three macronutrients without necessarily going overboard with the carbohydrates.

So, a good breakfast should still contain some carbohydrates, but that shouldn't be the center of the meal. You can definitely introduce food items such as egg whites (a single yolk mixed with lots of egg whites is fine) and dairy products.

You can eat white bread in the morning as long as you limit the quantity to one or two slices only. Remember: you still have the whole day ahead of you, so it's important that you don't go above your set carbohydrate limitation for the day.

Dairy products such as milk, cheese, and yogurt are part of a healthy PCOS diet. However, you should be careful of three things when buying dairy products: sodium content, sugar, and fat. Dairy products are essential because they are natural sources of calcium and iron.

However, the benefits that you get from these two minerals can be undermined by excess sodium, sugar, and fat. In order to avoid this disadvantage, try purchasing dairy products that are enriched but are sodium reduced and fat reduced.

This way, you will be able to fully enjoy the benefits of dairy products without necessarily exposing yourself to additional risks.

10.   The number of calories that should be removed from your daily caloric intake is called the caloric deficit. Women typically need fewer calories than men in order to function normally.

If you are presently overweight *and* have already been diagnosed with PCOS, then it is important that you begin shedding the excess poundage to decrease the impact of PCOS on your body. You have to set a caloric deficit goal every day so your weight loss will be consistent.

Your caloric intake per day should not increase just because you are exercising. On the contrary: the caloric deficit should be maintained to ensure that the weight comes off easily.

Now, I know that many women have difficulty with the idea of exercising *and* dieting at the same time because cravings and other problems surface almost immediately after a woman works out. One of the best solutions to this problem is to *split* the target caloric deficit between exercise and diet.

The recommended daily caloric deficit for weight loss is between 500 calories to a maximum of 1000 calories. Your total calories for the day should never go below 1200 calories – make this your minimum intake per day!

So, let us say that you want to have a caloric deficit of 500 calories per day. If we split that figure between the exercise and diet then we would come up with this: 250-calorie deficit from your diet and a 250-calorie deficit from exercising.

If we look at the caloric deficit goal in this manner, the whole process of losing weight will seem less hostile and more achievable, because there isn't so much pressure with exercise or diet. As long as you monitor your diet and exercise progress, you are bound to hit the target daily caloric deficit.

11.   Research work on PCOS is constantly evolving; professionals from both sides of the fence (conventional medicine and alternative healing) are working furiously to find possible aids for PCOS sufferers. Here are some noteworthy supplements and food items that have shown promise in terms of alleviating the symptoms of PCOS:

> The whole family of B vitamins have all shown promise in terms of normalizing the hormone levels in the female body.

You can easily get an adequate amount of B vitamins from quality multivitamin supplements, or you can just eat more green, leafy vegetables if you want to take a more natural route.

Whole grain cereals also contain B vitamins, so if you are able to eat lots of green, leafy vegetables and whole grain cereals on a daily basis, you won't have to worry about vitamin B deficiency at all.

If you are on any kind of medication at the moment, do consult with your physician first before purchasing any new supplement.

Most vitamin supplements are fine, even if the patient has diabetes or heart disease, but it's always better to speak to one's physician before adding anything to a current medical regimen.

> Hormone problems in women can lead to brittle bones, which may cause severe problems especially in senior ladies.

The most readily available source of calcium is cow's milk and other dairy products. If you are unable to tolerate dairy products, you can opt for a calcium supplement.

However, do keep in mind that in order for the body to be able to properly utilize calcium, you need to have adequate vitamin D levels in your body.

You can boost vitamin D levels in your body by eating fortified eggs, drinking fortified milk, or by exposing yourself to natural sunlight.

Vitamin D is not really a pre-requisite when it comes to absorbing calcium, but it really does help speed up the process.

Additionally, having sufficient vitamin D in your body will ensure that most of the calcium that you are taking in will be routed and stored in your bones, where the mineral is always needed.

> If you do not have any issues with dietary fiber, feel free to consume more in the coming days. Fiber doesn't really add anything t in terms of vitamins and minerals, but it is equally important (like water).

Fiber helps detoxify the body, and is also a key player when it comes to collecting and removing solid wastes from the large intestines.

Consuming a sufficient quantity of dietary fiber will also ensure that you will feel fuller for a longer period of time. Why is the feeling of fullness important for PCOS patients?

More often than not, PCOS patients feel hungry because they have to cut down on their sugars and carbs. It is very easy to give in to temptations if a person is unable to do something about the mad rumblings of her stomach.

The fastest way to solve this conundrum is by eating more fiber. Dietary fiber interacts with water, and also expands in the stomach and intestines.

When something occupies space in the digestive tract, the brain receives a signal that you are full and this, in turn, will dampen your appetite.

When you feel full, your brain will send a message that you should stop eating. As you can already imagine, this will be one of the easiest ways to tame a raging appetite, especially in the first few weeks of your new PCOS diet.

> Turmeric is one of the few herbal plants that are actually showing promise when doctors perform standard medical research. In lapidary tests, it has been shown that turmeric has a potent anti-inflammatory effect on the body, and it can actually help reduce blood sugar levels in the body.

> Vitamin E, or tocopherol, is also notable because it has a strong antioxidant effect on the body. Detoxification is essential for PCOS sufferers and a daily vitamin E pill just might help speed up the detox process.

Note, however, that you may only consume a maximum of 1 gram of vitamin E per day. Do not go above 1 gram/1000 milligrams as the excess vitamin E may cause other problems.

PCOS & Fertility Issues

One of the dire consequences of having polycystic ovarian syndrome is infertility, or the inability to conceive a child. If you have PCOS and have been having difficulties as of late, then know that you can still do something to improve your chances of conceiving. Below are some guidelines that you should keep in mind if you want to increase the chances of conceiving soon:

1. A woman's BMI has a large bearing on her ability to conceive. A large percentage of women with PCOS and upper body obesity experience some degree of difficulty in conceiving. The difficult in conceiving is often linked to hormonal issues that prevent obese PCOS patients from experiencing normal menstrual cycles.

   So, if you are overweight, one of your highest priorities right now is to lose weight. Don't despair though: medical science states that if you lose just ten pounds of body weight, your chances of conceiving goes up considerably.

   Ten pounds isn't much in the grand scale of things, but it helps the body tremendously in terms of rebalancing the natural hormone levels.

2. If you do conceive a child after you have been diagnosed with PCOS, you still have to be careful with your diet. Having hormonal issues often means that even the child in the womb is affected by how your body utilizes nutrients and calories.

   Without a sensible diet plan, you may experience giving birth too early (premature labor) or your child may become too big as he is developing inside the womb (this is caused by increased blood sugar levels throughout the gestation).

3. Inflammation inside the body should be avoided at all costs if you are trying to conceive. If you are trying to conceive, then it is imperative that you limit your consumption of pork and beef (red meats in general can cause some degree of inflammation at the cellular level). Chicken and fish should be the order of the day, though the fish may also need to be limited after you have already successfully conceived.

4. Even if you are not pregnant yet, current studies recommend that you begin taking folic acid supplements to help correct your ovulation cycle. Your daily folic acid goal is four hundred micrograms. Folic acid is present in green, leafy vegetables, seafood, and in enriched bread products.

Recommended Products:

1. PCOS Unlocked

2. Ovarian Cyst Miracle

References

Glycemic index and glycemic load for 100+ foods
http://www.health.harvard.edu/newsweek/Glycemic_index_
and_glycemic_load_for_100_foods.htm

GLYCEMIC INDEX and GLYCEMIC LOAD of COMMON FOODS
http://www.wellsource.org/8WW/updates/GI-GL-2p-
UsualServings.pdf

Glycemic index and glycemic load for 100+ foods
http://www.health.harvard.edu/newsweek/Glycemic_index_
and_glycemic_load_for_100_foods.htm

Polycystic Ovary Syndrome (PCOS) - Topic Overview
http://women.webmd.com/tc/polycystic-ovary-syndrome-
pcos-topic-overview

Polycystic Ovary Syndrome (PCOS) - Topic Overview
(continued)
http://women.webmd.com/tc/polycystic-ovary-syndrome-
pcos-cause

Polycystic Ovary Syndrome (PCOS) - Symptoms

http://women.webmd.com/tc/polycystic-ovary-syndrome-pcos-symptoms

Polycystic Ovary Syndrome (PCOS) - What Increases Your Risk
http://women.webmd.com/who-is-affected-by-polycystic-ovary-syndrome

Polycystic Ovary Syndrome (PCOS) - When To Call a Doctor
http://women.webmd.com/tc/polycystic-ovary-syndrome-pcos-when-to-call-adoctor

Conditions with symptoms similar to polycystic ovary syndrome (PCOS)
http://women.webmd.com/conditions-with-symptoms-similar-to-polycystic-ovarysyndrome-pcos

Polycystic Ovary Syndrome (PCOS) - Exams and Tests
http://women.webmd.com/tc/polycystic-ovary-syndrome-pcos-exams-and-tests

Polycystic Ovary Syndrome (PCOS) - Exams and Tests (Continued)
http://women.webmd.com/tc/polycystic-ovary-syndrome-pcos-exams-andtests?page=2

Polycystic Ovary Syndrome (PCOS) - Exams and Tests (Continued, pt. 3)
http://women.webmd.com/tc/polycystic-ovary-syndrome-pcos-exams-and-tests

Polycystic Ovary Syndrome (PCOS) - Treatment Overview

http://women.webmd.com/tc/polycystic-ovary-syndrome-pcos-treatment-overview

Polycystic Ovary Syndrome (PCOS) - Treatment Overview (continued)
http://women.webmd.com/tc/polycystic-ovary-syndrome-pcos-treatmentoverview?page=2

Polycystic Ovary Syndrome (PCOS) - Medications
http://women.webmd.com/tc/polycystic-ovary-syndrome-pcos-medications

Healthy Diet for Polycystic Ovary Syndrome - Topic Overview
http://women.webmd.com/tc/healthy-diet-for-polycystic-ovary-syndrome-topic-overview

PCOS DIET STUDIES
http://www.livestrong.com/article/249273-pcos-diet-studies/#ixzz2esRIPnXM

ORGANIC PCOS DIET
http://www.livestrong.com/article/534141-organic-pcos-diet/#ixzz2esRKilQF

PCOS DIET PLANS
ttp://www.livestrong.com/article/399988-pcos-diet-plans/#ixzz2esRiwy1x

FOODS FOR A PCOS DIET
http://www.livestrong.com/article/190388-foods-for-a-pcos-diet/#ixzz2esS0eth6

PCOS & LOW GLYCEMIC DIET

http://www.livestrong.com/article/226671-pcos-low-glycemic-diet/#ixzz2esS5B2Ki

PCOS AND ACNE DIET
http://www.livestrong.com/article/207724-pcos-and-acne-diet/#ixzz2esSAeWOd

PCOS & PALEO DIET
http://www.livestrong.com/article/550003-pcos-paleo-diet/#ixzz2esSF43Ep

RECOMMENDED DIET FOR PCOS
http://www.livestrong.com/article/199992-recommended-diet-for-pcos/#ixzz2esSJENlf

LOW GLYCEMIC-LOAD DIET FOR PCOS
http://www.livestrong.com/article/217800-low-glycemic-load-diet-for-pcos/#ixzz2esSTOqBV

LOW GI DIET FOR PCOS
http://www.livestrong.com/article/358474-low-gi-diet-for-pcos/#ixzz2esSXlHqh

1200 CALORIE DIET FOR PCOS
http://www.livestrong.com/article/410231-1200-calorie-diet-for-pcos/#ixzz2esSbrTrz

THE BEST DIET FOR WOMEN WITH PCOS
http://www.livestrong.com/article/527704-the-best-diet-for-women-with-pcos/#ixzz2esSfzrAp

DIET TO HELP CONTROL PCOS
http://www.livestrong.com/article/358776-diet-to-help-control-pcos/#ixzz2esSjYlHC

DIET FOR PCOS AND INSULIN RESISTANCE
http://www.livestrong.com/article/345227-diet-for-pcos-and-insulin-resistance/#ixzz2esSnCZf8

GRAIN-FREE DIET FOR PCOS
http://www.livestrong.com/article/418637-grain-free-diet-for-pcos/#ixzz2esSs8OMj

HOW TO LOSE WEIGHT WITH PCOS
http://www.livestrong.com/article/215361-how-to-lose-weight-fast-with-pcos/#ixzz2esTCHnDg

HCG DIET TO TREAT PCOS
http://www.livestrong.com/article/535835-hcg-diet-to-treat-pcos/#ixzz2esTH6Mn8

WHAT TO EAT WHEN YOU HAVE PCOS?
http://www.livestrong.com/article/445892-what-to-eat-when-you-have-pcos/#ixzz2esTK7SpL

A LOW CARB DIET FOR PCOS SYMPTOMS
http://www.livestrong.com/article/347395-a-low-carb-diet-for-pcos-symptoms/#ixzz2esTNqpZa

PCOS WEIGHT LOSS PLANS
http://www.livestrong.com/article/418499-pcos-weight-loss-plans/#ixzz2esTXebN1

VEGETARIAN DIET FOR PCOS
http://www.livestrong.com/article/366467-vegetarian-diet-for-pcos/#ixzz2esTaqFs5

CAFFEINE & POLYCYSTIC OVARIES

http://www.livestrong.com/article/541151-caffeine-polycystic-ovaries/#ixzz2esTeFjyT

LIST OF FOODS PCOS SUFFERERS CAN'T EAT
http://www.livestrong.com/article/71425-list-foods-pcos-sufferers-cant/#ixzz2esThxvj2

PCOS DIET AND PREGNANCY
http://www.livestrong.com/article/426013-pcos-diet-and-pregnancy/

PCOS DIET TO GET PREGNANT
http://www.livestrong.com/article/366574-pcos-diet-to-get-pregnant/#ixzz2esRMwwLk

THE PCOS DIET FOR FERTILITY
http://www.livestrong.com/article/358989-the-pcos-diet-for-fertility/#ixzz2esRUAxUS

NATURAL DIET FOR PCOS & INFERTILITY
http://www.livestrong.com/article/228163-natural-diet-for-pcos-infertility/#ixzz2esRtypfS